5 Justifications for Why You Ought to Begin Utilizing natural skincare items

NZEKWE EMMANUEL

5 Justifications for Why You Ought to Begin Utilizing natural skincare items

ISBN:9798353194101

DEDICATION

I dedicate this book to almighty God.

CONTENTS

ACKNOWLEDGMENTS

I sincerely thank God the Almighty for his grace, provisions and love in my life and throughout my time in writing this book.

Chapter one

Organic Items Are Really great for the Climate

A great deal of those non-natural cosmetics and other corrective things you're accustomed to utilizing are quite terrible for the climate. Making non-natural items requires plants that produce vapor and poisonous gasses.

They will more often than exclude mixtures like oil,

aluminum and lead, a significant number of which require mining and don't play especially well when left in land-fills. Aluminum mining in especially is an extremely perilous and unrewarding position, that has been known to cause malignant growth and Alzheimer's for quite a while. Numerous other unsafe substances will likewise track down their direction back into the biological system through different means.

Aside from the way that this is awful for the specialists, it can likewise be cruel on the climate that is being drained dry of its regular assets.

It's anything but an industry you ought to fundamentally be supporting!

Alternately, natural items use fixings that come from regular cultivating and natural planting. These are items that are made by working with the land, and obviously, they're incredibly great for the planet.

Also, don't even get us going on creature testing.

CHAPTER TWO

They Do Exclude Brutal Synthetic compounds

What will at first draw in the vast majority to natural cosmetics and skincare however, is the opportunity it manages the cost of them from brutal synthetics. These items incorporate a ton of possibly hurtful fixings and these incorporate any semblance of parabens and phthalates, which have been connected to disease and type 2 diabetes among different issues.

Indeed, even where this isn't true, frequently the unnatural smells and restricting specialists involved can cause a scope of responses in the skin, prompting rashes and more issues.

Insufficient for you? Here are only a couple of different fixings tossed into our sun blocks, creams, and concealers:

Lead: Lead was eliminated from school pencils because of how much wellbeing concerns encompassing it and the high probability that it is cancer-causing. In spite of this, lead is as yet utilized in huge amounts in various cosmetics.

Parfum: Parfum isn't only one item yet a term that incorporates a wide range of items. These are intended to add aroma to our skincare items (since that is important?) as well as things prefer cleansing agents. They can cause a tremendous scope of issues going from rashes, to migraines, to dazedness, to skin staining.

Believe it or not, the organization delivering the items expected to further develop your skin is effectively adding fixings that can harm its tone and make rashes. So it will smell pleasant. Go figure!

Aluminum: Nothing bad can be said about aluminum on a fundamental level, it's the point at which you apply everything over your skin that it turns into an issue! Aluminum is tracked down in antiperspirants specifically, however can be found somewhere else as well. This has estrogen-like impacts, which can harm your chemical equilibrium, prompting loss of bulk, melancholy, from there, the sky is the limit.

Estrogenic Mixtures: Discussing which, there are quite numerous estrogenic mixtures in cosmetics and skin items, that their removal through the sewers has really prompted the normal male's testosterone levels dropping fundamentally.

What to be aware before you take a stab at utilizing these items is that the skin will retain anything that you put on it. This implies that those fixings will ultimately advance toward your circulatory system and that is where large numbers of the more difficult issues originate from.

Perilous Synthetic compounds Utilized in Customary Cleanser

In addition to your cosmetics and skincare items contain these impurities and poisons all things considered! Think about cleanser...

Strolling around with strong synthetic substances in your hair is - obviously - not particularly great for you. This implies you'll be engrossing those synthetic substances through your skin and furthermore breathing in the vapor.

Obviously the gamble this includes relies upon the item you've picked however the inquiry you need to pose is -

do you trust the makers to have done all necessary investigation?

One thing we do be aware, is that numerous shampoos and conditions really contain engineered estrogen compounds. As referenced, these work very much like genuine estrogens and can really keep the body from delivering the perfect proportion of testosterone.

Low testosterone is a portion of a plague among men right now and this is much of the time remembered to be one reason why. Assuming that you utilize manufactured shampoos, this could add to low state of mind, low energy, weight gain and possibly even fruitlessness!

These are a few very valid justifications to change to natural shampoos. Then, at that point, there are the additional advantages you get from picking one of the most mind-blowing natural conditioner choices - you'll furnish your scalp and hair with additional regular oils and supplements for example to help better in general wellbeing, you'll furnish yourself with a more wonderful normal fragrance and you'll try and have the option to profit from getting the items a lot less expensive much of the time!

What is Fluoride?

What about toothpaste?

Fluoride is remembered for most toothpastes and we're much of the time told that it tends to be an extremely powerful device in fighting cavities. While this may to be sure be valid, what we catch wind of less frequently is that it can likewise cause an enormous number of issues.

That is on the grounds that fluoride is poisonous and in high dosages it can really harm your teeth. It might try and be connected with learning inabilities.

Still not persuaded about fluoride? Then consider that the main approach to making fluoride is really to extricate it from the airborne modern waste radiated by compost producers? Decent.

Presently this is where things get fascinating, in light of the fact that you see fluoride is quite in our water. States chose for add it there, accepting that it would assist with working on our teeth and eliminate microorganisms.

This steamed a many individuals as you might have expected and simultaneously it implies that you truly don't require it added to your toothpaste! There's all that could possibly be needed of it in the water as of now for any constructive outcomes to be appreciated.

Gracious and coincidentally, fluoride is neurotoxic implying that it really causes cerebrum harm!

CHAPTER THREE

They Are Wealthy in Supplements and Smell Perfect

Natural items don't contain everything and hence won't hurt your skin.

A long way from hurting your skin as a matter of fact, these natural cosmetics items will give you a lot of normal supplements including nutrients, minerals and amino acids.

Once more, these are consumed into the body and they can be utilized to make you look more brilliant in the long haul as well as the short. Frequently these even incorporate regular cell reinforcements, which can safeguard your skin cells and forestall untimely maturing - as well as fighting off disease!

Here is what to perceive: your body advanced in nature. We advanced to flourish in our common habitats, and in this way we are actually intended to profit from the supplements that come from the mud, the plants, and the ocean. At the point when you apply those to your face, it resembles returning home again for your body. It's fantastic for you.

Goodness and regular cosmetics additionally smell perfect and feel much improved. Rather than being, brutal, tacky and chemicalsmelling, they'll be delicate, saturating and regular. Some of them even taste very great…

CHAPTER FOUR

They Are Tomfoolery and Individual

Like all that wasn't sufficient, regular cosmetics is only loads of tomfoolery and it's profoundly fulfilling. Envision this discussion:

"Pleasant lipstick!"

"Much obliged, I made it myself!"

How remunerating could that be? What's more, when you let them know it's custom made, natural lipstick, it will undoubtedly prompt an extraordinary discussion.

At the point when you make your own natural cosmetics, you can make your ideal shade, feel and tone. Furthermore, you know it will have a really inconspicuous and regular tint since it is produced using truly normal and unpretentious fixings.

We really gained our concept of what's 'delightful' from our time spent in the wild when we were advancing. So assuming that you look more normal, you will show up naturally more lovely...

CHAPTER FIVE

They're Modest!

With such countless valid justifications to change to natural items, you're likely thinking about what the catch is. It should be the cost right?

Not a chance! The cost is maybe the best piece. Numerous natural items - as you'll realize when you read the full digital book - can be made as effectively as blending a few things in your cabinet. This implies there's no outing to the grocery store fundamental, and you can begin helping immediately.

That, however it will save you Truckload of cash. Also, regardless of whether you choose to purchase natural items, instead of make them, they're as yet less expensive than the engineered other options!

There is in a real sense not a glaringly obvious

explanation not to trade.

ABOUT THE AUTHOR

As the son of a french father and East European mother, Emmanuel Sees himself as a world citizen and galactic being who speaks the universal language of the soul. Emmanuel Always knew that there is more to life than meets the eye or what society teaches us.
USA today selling author Nzekwe Emmanuel, Engineer by the day , author by night who pens adventurous and edgy romance stories by the light of his smart phone flash light app.

5 Justifications for Why You Ought to Begin Utilizing natural skincare items

5 Justifications for Why You Ought to Begin Utilizing natural skincare items

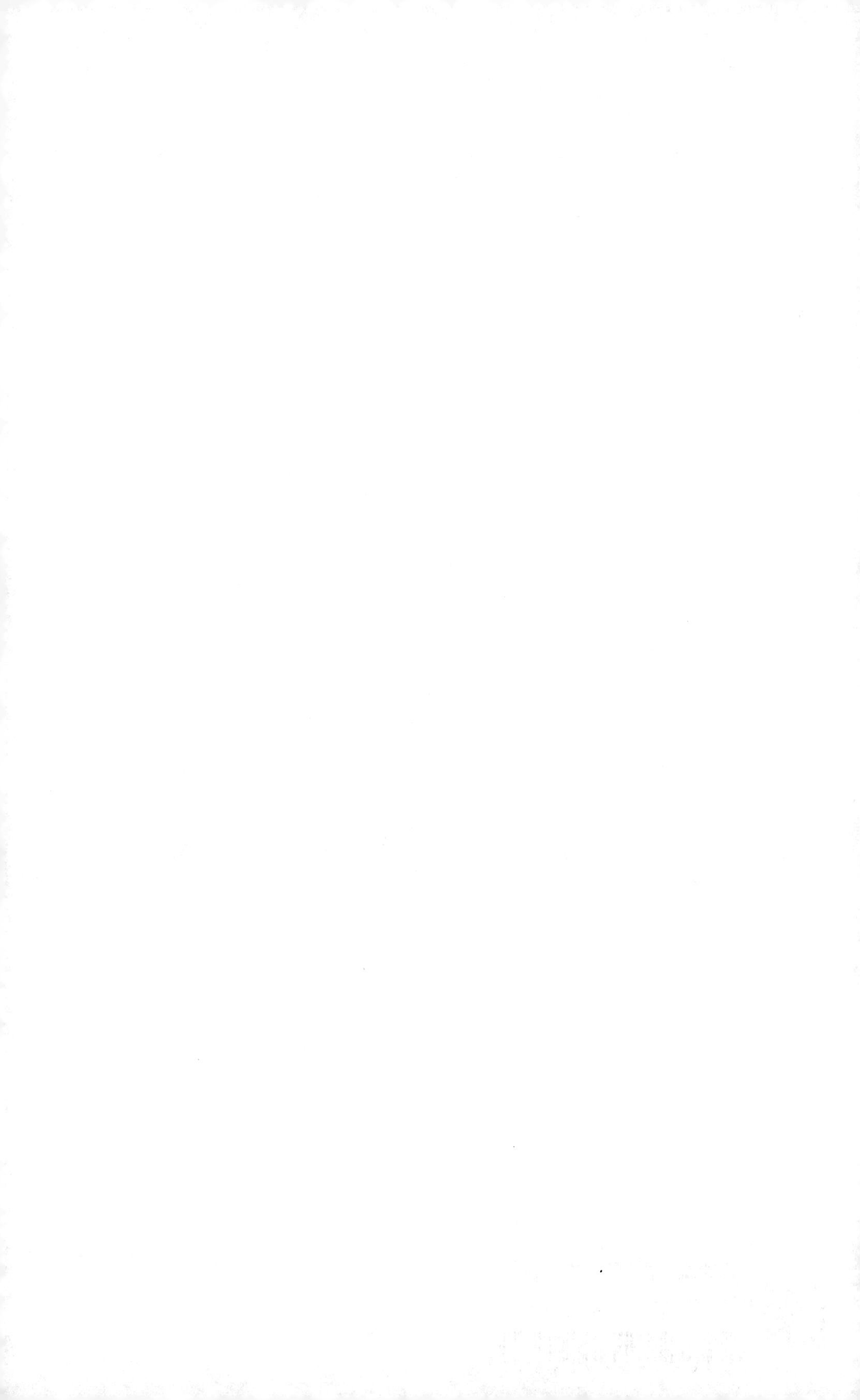

www.ingramcontent.com/pod-product-compliance
Lightning Source LLC
LaVergne TN
LVHW020546160826
845677LV00015B/4232
9798353194101